HERBAL HEMORRHAGE CONTROL

Empower Your Health, Harnessing Techniques For Nature's Healing Touch

DR. JEREMY ALLEY

Disclaimer:

The information provided in this book, is intended for general informational purposes only and should not be considered as professional advice.

The author has made every effort to ensure the accuracy of the information presented. However, readers are advised to consult with a qualified healthcare professional before attempting any herbal remedies or making significant changes to their wellness routine. Individual health conditions vary, and what may be suitable for one person may not be appropriate for another.

It is important to note that the author is not in any endorsement deal, partnership, or affiliation with any organization, brand, or company mentioned in this book. Any references to specific products or services are based on the author's personal experience or general knowledge and do not imply an endorsement or promotion of those products or services.

Contents

Overview

We explore the profound benefits of nature's healing abilities as we dig into the world of herbal medicines for wound healing and hemorrhage control in this complete book. Across many cultures, herbal remedies have been used for generations to promote overall wellness. As we set out on our adventure, we will reveal the knowledge ingrained in customs and illuminate the possibility of using herbs to aid in healing and avoid difficulties.

About The Book

Welcome to a comprehensive investigation of herbal treatments for wound healing and bleeding prevention.

This guide is designed to give alternative treatments that capitalize on the power of medicinal plants, as well as insightful information on the field of natural health. We cordially welcome you to explore the ancient knowledge that herbal treatments offer to the field of wound care and bleeding control.

The Book's Objective

This book aims to provide readers with a thorough grasp of herbal treatments as effective means of controlling bleeding and repairing wounds. By exploring the medicinal qualities of many herbs, we hope to arm readers with information that can supplement traditional medical practices. This book is a resource to help you make well-informed decisions for your health, regardless of whether you're looking for alternatives or are just interested in learning more about the possibilities of herbal remedies.

How Herbal Remedies Can Help Control Hemorrhage and Promote Wound Healing

Traditional medicine has relied heavily on herbal medicines because of their proven ability to reduce bleeding and promote wound healing. This section delves into the methods by which plants apply their therapeutic effects. Herbs have several uses when it comes to treating wounds, from encouraging tissue regeneration to having antibacterial and anti-inflammatory properties. We also explore the function of herbs in hemorrhage management, looking at their potential to promote blood coagulation and lessen severe bleeding. Knowing the science underlying herbal treatments helps us appreciate these natural remedies and how important a role they may play in holistic wellness.

CHAPTER ONE

COMPREHENDING INJURIES

A person may sustain wounds as a result of trauma, accidents, or surgical operations. Their intensity and nature can differ, necessitating the use of various strategies to promote appropriate healing and avoid problems. Comprehending the characteristics of injuries is essential for executing efficient care and therapy.

Kinds Of Injuries

There are many different types of wounds, and each one presents different care and treatment concerns. Abrasions are superficial skin injuries that are frequently brought on by scraping or rubbing on an uneven surface. Deeper cuts or tears in the skin, typically brought on by sharp instruments, are called lacerations. When a sharp item pierces the skin, it can introduce hazardous microorganisms, resulting in puncture wounds. Intentional cuts performed during medical operations result in surgical wounds, which require specific care to promote recovery.

The Process Of Wound Healing

The goal of the intricate and dynamic wound healing process is to repair damaged tissues back to their original state. The proliferative, maturation, and inflammatory phases are the three main stages that it usually goes through.

Phase of Inflammation: The body's initial reaction to the damage occurs during this phase. To reduce bleeding, blood arteries narrow, and platelets create a temporary plug at the site of the wound. As inflammation develops, white blood cells are drawn to the location to help clear debris and protect against infection.

Phase of Proliferation: In this phase, new tissue grows to replace the damaged area. One type of cell called fibroblasts is essential for the production of collagen, the structural protein that serves as the basis for scar tissue. Additionally, blood arteries enlarge to carry nutrients and oxygen to the growing tissue.

Phase of Maturation: The last stage concentrates on reshaping the just-created tissue.

The scar tissue is further refined and extra collagen is broken down. The scar that results from this procedure may gradually disappear over months or years.

Investigating holistic strategies for wound healing that encourage recuperation and reduce complications is crucial.

Herbal treatments are complementary to or substitutes for traditional wound care techniques because of their ability to promote the body's innate healing mechanisms.

Since they have a wide range of medicinal benefits, herbs have long been used in traditional medical systems. Certain herbs are thought to have antibacterial, anti-inflammatory, and tissue-regenerating properties that aid in wound healing.

These herbs could consist of:

Calendula: Applied topically to wounds, calendula's anti-inflammatory and antibacterial qualities aid in the healing process and lessen inflammation.

Aloe Vera: Known for its calming and cooling properties, aloe vera is frequently used to reduce pain and hasten the healing process for wounds, burns, and abrasions.

Comfrey: Due to its ability to regenerate cells, comfrey has been utilized traditionally. It might lessen inflammation and help wounds heal.

Lavender: The calming scent and antibacterial qualities of lavender essential oil are well-known. When administered topically and diluted, it might aid in the healing of wounds.

Chamomile: Chamomile has antioxidant and anti-inflammatory qualities. Because of its delicate nature, it can be used on minor wounds and sensitive skin.

Herbal Treatment For Hemorrhage

Herbs can be investigated for their capacity to control hemorrhage or excessive bleeding in addition to their ability to heal wounds. It's thought that several herbs have hemostatic qualities that help to stop bleeding and encourage clotting.

Yarrow: Yarrow has long been used to encourage blood coagulation and halt bleeding. Because of its astringent qualities, it may be able to help treat small cuts and wounds.

Capsaicin-rich cayenne pepper is believed to increase blood flow and aid in clotting. It can be applied topically or moderately ingested due to its possible hemostatic properties.

Witch Hazel: Witch hazel has an astringent quality that may help constrict and tighten blood vessels, assisting in the control of bleeding.

Herbal medicines can be quite helpful in controlling bleeding and aiding in wound healing, but they must be used carefully.

The appropriate identification of herbs, safety concerns, and advice from medical experts should all be taken into account when using them. Including herbal remedies in a thorough wound care plan can help create a more all-encompassing strategy that encourages the body's natural healing mechanisms.

CHAPTER TWO

HERBS FOR HEALING WONDERS

Injuries and wounds are a part of life, and it makes sense to look for natural solutions to speed up their healing.

It has been demonstrated that several herbs are useful in accelerating wound healing and reducing bleeding. Aloe Vera is a notable participant among these.

Aloe Vera: The Plant Of Healing By Nature

Aloe Vera, sometimes known as "nature's healing plant," is well known for its extraordinary ability to heal wounds.

Numerous bioactive substances found in the gel made from its succulent leaves aid in tissue repair and lessen inflammation. Aloe Vera gel used directly on wounds can reduce discomfort and hasten the healing process.

Utilization Of Wound Healing Application

Using a variety of techniques, the application of herbal medicines for wound healing focuses on utilizing the medicinal qualities of particular plants. For example, aloe vera gel can be applied directly to wounds to be utilized topically.

Aloe Vera Gel Production

The procedure of making aloe vera gel at home is easy. Slice open the leaf to release the gel, then take a scoop and apply it to the wound. This organic gel serves as an infection-prevention barrier in addition to hastening the healing process.

Calendula: The Herbal Antiseptic

Calendula is well known for its ability to soothe skin and is another herb with strong wound-healing capabilities. This vivid orange flower is frequently used to treat cuts, bruises, and other skin irritations. There are several ways to use calendula for wound treatment.

Applying Calendula Oil Topically

The petals of the plant are used to make calendula oil, which is topically applied to wounds. Its antibacterial and anti-inflammatory qualities help to stop infections and lessen swelling.

Applying calendula oil to wounds regularly encourages quicker healing and reduces scarring.

Internal Use Of Calendula Tea

Calendula can be drunk as tea internally. Internal intake enhances general health by enhancing the body's immune response and facilitating the healing process from the inside, even though it might not directly treat surface lesions.

Known by many as the "knit bone" plant, comfrey has been used traditionally to aid in the healing of bones and tissues. Allantoin, a substance recognized for its capacity to regenerate cells, is present in this herb.

Poultice of Comfrey

Making a poultice using comfrey is one efficient technique to use for wound healing. Crushing or combining comfrey leaves into a paste and applying it directly to the wound is the process of making a poultice. This can hasten the healing process for bruises, wounds, and scrapes.

Craft a Comfrey Salve

You can make a comfrey salve for a more practical application. Beeswax and oil infused with comfrey are combined to make a salve that can be kept and used as needed. This salve minimizes scarring, encourages tissue regeneration, and acts as a barrier of defense.

Using these herbal medicines in conjunction with wound care can be a comprehensive and all-natural strategy for encouraging healing and avoiding infections. But speaking with a medical expert is crucial, particularly in cases of serious injuries or chronic illnesses.

CHAPTER THREE

HERBAL MEDICATIONS FOR CONTROLLING HEMORRHAGE

Excessive bleeding, also known as hemorrhage, is a medical emergency that needs to be treated right away. Knowing the nature of bleeding, its varieties, and how to gauge its intensity are crucial when investigating herbal remedies for bleeding management.

Recognizing Hemorrhage

Blood can leak out of the circulatory system either internally or externally, which is known as hemorrhage.

While external bleeding is noticeable, internal bleeding may not be as obvious, making identification more difficult. Whichever kind it is, early management is essential to avoid consequences.

Different Types Of Bleeding

Hemorrhage comes in several forms, and each needs to be managed with a different strategy. Because arteries have a higher pressure, arterial bleeding, which is characterized by brilliant red, spurting blood, requires immediate medical attention. Significant venous hemorrhage also has darker, more consistent blood flow. Although it is usually not as severe, capillary bleeding can persist.

Identifying The Level Of Bleeding

Determining the extent of bleeding is an essential ability. While minor bleeding can be controlled with first aid alone, significant bleeding necessitates emergency medical treatment.

Severe bleeding symptoms include weakness, fast blood loss, and a drop in blood pressure. Knowing these signs enables you to choose the right herbal cure.

Yarrow: The Hemostatic of Nature

There is a long history of using yarrow (Achillea millefolium) as a hemostatic plant, which can stop bleeding. Its astringent qualities play a role in vasoconstriction and clot formation. Yarrow can be taken internally in a variety of forms or applied topically.

A Tincture Of Yarrow For Emergencies

An effective treatment for controlling bleeding in an emergency is yarrow tincture, which is prepared by steeping yarrow in alcohol. When applied directly onto wounds, it reduces blood loss and promotes blood coagulation. This tincture offers a rapid and effective solution to unexpected bleeding, making it an invaluable addition to any first aid box.

Yarrow Tea as an Internal Remedy

You can drink yarrow tea internally. In addition to aiding the body's natural clotting processes, the tea's anti-inflammatory qualities help lessen the discomfort and swelling brought on by bleeding. Frequent consumption may improve circulatory health in general.

Cayenne Pepper: An Effective Herb for Circulation

The benefits of cayenne pepper (Capsicum annum) on the circulatory system are well known. It has capsaicin, which has vasodilatory properties and increases blood circulation, supporting normal blood flow. Cayenne is essential for controlling blood pressure when it comes to preventing bleeding.

A poultice of Cayenne Pepper

Wounds can be externally treated with a poultice comprised of cayenne pepper and a base, such as coconut oil or olive oil. By increasing blood flow to the injured area, the poultice promotes healing and reduces bleeding. This technique is especially helpful for wounds that continue to bleed.

Adding cayenne to the diet daily can benefit circulatory health in addition to its immediate first aid benefits. Cayenne helps the body stop and regulate bleeding, whether it's taken as a supplement or added to food.

Herbal treatments for bleeding control, such as yarrow and cayenne pepper, are beneficial. However, before choosing the best course of action, it's critical to assess the type and extent of bleeding.

When used sparingly, these herbs can be effective allies in supporting healthy circulation and supporting the body's inherent healing mechanisms.

CHAPTER FOUR

ACCESSORY PRACTICES

Complementary therapies are essential for wound healing and bleeding control. This section explores several methods that enhance the efficacy of herbal remedies in aiding in healing. Readers can learn about a comprehensive approach to recovery that goes beyond the technical parts of treatment, such as stress management and mindfulness practices.

Appropriate Clotting Techniques

Taking care of wounds properly is one of the essential components in encouraging healing. This chapter describes the basic procedures for wound care and looks at how these procedures can be easily incorporated with the use of herbal remedies. Readers will acquire important insights on creating the best possible environment for the body's natural healing processes, from cleaning to dressing practices.

Sanitizing and disinfecting

Keeping the wound clean and sterile is essential to avoiding infections and encouraging a quick recovery. This section explores the role that cleanliness plays in wound care and offers several herbal remedies that can help with the disinfection process. Readers can promote their general well-being by being proactive and realizing the role that cleanliness plays in healing.

Clothes Methods

An important part of the healing process is selecting the appropriate dressing for a wound. This chapter looks at several methods of dressing and how to use herbal remedies in these methods. Readers will learn useful tips for maximizing the healing environment by using the right dressing techniques, regardless of the severity of the wounds.

Food for the Healing of Wounds

Beyond medical attention from outside sources, diet is essential for promoting the body's healing processes. The significance of a balanced diet in accelerating wound healing is emphasized in this section. The function of vital nutrients and how herbal remedies can supplement food choices to improve the healing process overall will be explained to readers.

Minerals and Vitamins

The body's capacity to repair is significantly influenced by specific vitamins and minerals. This chapter highlights herbal sources that are rich in these necessary components and examines the particular nutrients that aid in wound healing. Readers may assist their healing process by making educated decisions by knowing the dietary aspects of healing.

Remedy Foods

Beyond conventional treatments, herbal remedies can also include therapeutic foods that promote healing and speed up the healing process. This section introduces readers to a range of foods that have natural healing qualities while highlighting the link between nutrition and health.

This chapter examines the culinary application of herbal remedies for wound healing and bleeding control, ranging from herbs to nutrient-dense choices.

Initially Aid Procedures

Everyone should be able to perform first aid on wounds as it is an essential skill. Understanding how to react to injuries quickly and efficiently can have a big impact on how quickly they heal.

The fundamentals of first aid for wounds are covered in this part, with a focus on the significance of prompt and proper action.

The first thing to do when a wound appears is to evaluate the situation and make sure the first responder and the victim are both safe. The three main components of basic first aid for wounds are wound cleanliness, bleeding control, and infection prevention. Comprehending these essential ideas lays the groundwork for providing efficient wound care.

Sanitizing and sterilizing wounds

To avoid infections and encourage the best possible healing, proper cleaning and disinfection are essential. This topic explores the significance of cleaning wounds with sterile solutions and mild antiseptics.

It also sheds light on the meticulous yet gentle methods needed to clean the wounded area of debris and strange objects.

Applying Makeup And Bandages

Using the proper bandages and dressings is essential to wound care. This section talks about the different kinds of dressings, like sticky bandages and sterile gauze, and stresses how important it is to select the best one for the type and severity of the wound. Also taught are the proper bandaging methods for providing support and securing dressings.

Essential Herbal First Aid Kit Items

Adding herbs to your first aid bag can speed up the healing process and provide all-natural substitutes for pharmaceutical therapies. This section examines the components of a herbal first aid kit, with a focus on choosing herbs that are recognized to have therapeutic benefits. These herbs, which range from the calming calendula to the antibacterial tea tree oil, are essential for encouraging the healing of wounds.

Essential Herbs For Fast Reaction

Some herbs are particularly effective in treating particular aspects of wound care, such as decreasing inflammation or speeding up the regeneration of tissue. This article explores the qualities of essential herbs to have on hand for emergency preparedness. Among the herbal heroes mentioned are chamomile, which has anti-inflammatory qualities, and lavender, which has relaxing benefits.

How To Make A Herbal First Aid Kit

Creating a customized herbal first-aid pack is a proactive step toward natural recovery. This section walks you through putting your kit together, stressing the value of accessibility and organization in times of need. With items like arnica for bruising and aloe vera gel for burns, your customized herbal first aid kit turns into a flexible tool for a range of circumstances.

CHAPTER FIVE

LIFESTYLE AND PREVENTION

Keeping your skin healthy is essential to avoiding sores and enhancing your general well-being.

A barrier that protects the skin naturally from injuries and diseases is healthy skin.

Maintaining the skin's cleanliness, moisture, and protection from damaging environmental elements are all part of a good skincare regimen.

 Frequent cleaning aids in the removal of bacteria and debris that may exacerbate wounds, particularly following physical exertion.

Dietary Advice for Skin Health is essential for both wound prevention and quick recovery.

A diet high in vitamins and minerals promotes skin resilience and regeneration.

Including foods rich in antioxidants, zinc, vitamin C, and vitamin E encourages the synthesis of collagen and fortifies the epidermis.

It is impossible to emphasize how crucial being hydrated is to preserving the health of your skin. Skin is robust and supple when the body is properly hydrated.

By flushing out toxins, improving circulation, decreasing skin dryness, and lowering the risk of cuts and cracks, drinking enough water helps.

The term "Lifestyle Practices to Prevent Wounds" refers to a variety of behaviors that improve general health.

Injury risk can be considerably decreased by avoiding extended exposure to severe temperatures, using protective clothing when engaging in physical activity, and exercising caution when in unknown places.

Frequent exercise enhances blood circulation, which supports the health of the skin.

Taking Care Of Your Feet: Athletes And Active People

The higher risk of injury in athletes and active individuals needs special attention to foot care. It's important to select footwear that fits properly and offers adequate support.

It is possible to intervene early and avoid consequences by routinely checking the feet for any indications of discomfort, blisters, or cuts.

Identifying And Managing Risk Factors

Being aware of the unique risk factors associated with wounds is crucial for preventative action. Chronic illnesses that affect the immune system, diabetes, or vascular diseases can weaken the skin's barrier function and make it more vulnerable to wounds.

Those who are aware of these risk factors can take the appropriate safety measures and, if necessary, consult a doctor. Those with underlying medical conditions must have regular check-ups and discussions with healthcare providers.

CHAPTER SIX

CASE RESEARCH

Examining real-world situations is crucial to comprehend the efficacy of herbal wound healing remedies and bleeding prevention. These case studies offer an in-depth look at a range of situations, including the kinds of wounds, how herbal treatments are applied, and the results that follow.

Through examining these experiences, people can learn how to use herbal remedies in a variety of contexts and develop a better grasp of their potential advantages.

Actual Success Stories

Success tales attest to the effectiveness of herbal remedies for wound healing. These personal accounts detail the experiences of people who have effectively treated bleeding and accelerated wound healing with herbal treatments.

These tales provide hope for the efficacy of herbal remedies while also providing useful information about the particular herbs and methods that worked in each particular situation. Success tales from real-world experiences help to expand the body of knowledge regarding herbal remedies for bleeding injuries.

Journeys For Healing Wounds

Setting out on a wound-healing journey requires a comprehensive strategy that goes beyond applying herbal medicines right away.

This section delves into the holistic approach to healing, taking into account elements like mental health, modifying lifestyle, and incorporating herbal remedies into daily activities. Experiences with recovering from wounds emphasize the value of perseverance and consistency while illuminating the complex process of rehabilitation. People can develop a deeper comprehension of the long-term advantages of herbal remedies in the healing process by looking at these travels.

Controlling Hemorrhage In Emergencies

The capacity to manage bleeding is crucial in emergency scenarios requiring quick action.

This section explores the herbal medicines and techniques that can be used to effectively manage bleeding during emergencies.

This section of the conversation offers helpful tips for using herbal remedies for effective and quick bleeding control, from recognizing herbs with coagulant qualities to knowing the right application techniques.

Those looking for natural first aid and quick response options must understand the role that herbs can play in emergencies.

Together, these parts add to a thorough grasp of the topic of herbal wound healing and hemorrhage management by fusing theoretical knowledge with real-world applications and experiences. This examination of these topics is ongoing.

CHAPTER SEVEN

AVOIDANCE AND RECOMMENDATIONS

It's important to know about potential dangers and contraindications before starting any herbal therapeutic path.

To ensure that herbal treatments are taken properly and with a full understanding of their potential consequences, this chapter discusses the safety precautions people should take.

Since safety is of the utmost importance, this section attempts to offer precise instructions for a safe herbal healing experience.

Recognizing Possible Dangers

Even while herbal remedies are usually regarded as safe, it is important to be informed of any possible hazards.

This chapter examines any negative reactions or side effects that could arise from using herbal remedies for fungal infections and athlete's foot. People can address any concerns about using herbal treatments and make educated decisions by being aware of these risks.

Speaking With Medical Experts

Collaboration between herbal remedies and conventional healthcare is key to comprehensive well-being.

The significance of speaking with medical professionals before beginning any herbal treatment is emphasized in this section.

These consultations guarantee that people receive tailored guidance and can successfully incorporate herbal remedies into their overall health plan.

This chapter provides practical safety tips for incorporating herbal medicine into daily life. From dosage recommendations to storage guidelines, readers will gain valuable insights on how to maximize the benefits of herbal remedies while maintaining a safe and sustainable approach to health and wellness.

CONCLUSION

As we wrap up the exploration of herbal solutions for athlete's foot and fungal infections, it's essential to summarize key takeaways and insights gained throughout the book.

This conclusion serves as a reflection on the potential impact of herbal remedies, emphasizing their role in holistic well-being.

Recap Of Herbal Solutions

A concise recapitulation of the herbal solutions discussed serves as a quick reference for readers. This section highlights the key herbs, their benefits, and application methods, providing a comprehensive summary for those who want to revisit specific remedies or concepts.

Encouragement For Readers On Their Healing Journey

The healing journey is unique for each individual. This final section offers words of encouragement, motivating readers to embark on their healing journey with confidence.

By incorporating herbal solutions into their daily lives, individuals can take proactive steps toward managing and preventing athlete's foot and fungal infections, fostering a healthier and more balanced lifestyle.

this book serves as a comprehensive guide to herbal solutions for athlete's foot and fungal infections.

By understanding the nature of these conditions and exploring the benefits of herbal remedies, readers are equipped with valuable knowledge to enhance their well-being naturally.